THE ALPHA MEAL

MAXIMIZING FITNESS, PERFORMANCE & WELLNESS WITH THE MOST IMPORTANT MEAL OF THE DAY.

BRANDON MENTORE

Acknowledgements:

To my family and friends who have always supported my pursuit of knowledge.

About the author:

Brandon Mentore has worked in the health and fitness industry for 20 years. Acquiring a degree in health and exercise sciences was merely the first step in his pursuit of understanding human health and biology. Taking advanced courses, studying countless hours and acquiring multiple certifications he has become fluent in virtually all aspects of health and fitness. Not only does he personally work with clients to engineer personal health programs he's an expert consultant, speaker, educator and writer appearing in over 100 publications on line and in print for outlets such as CNN, Mensfitness, Mensjournal, Shape and Huffington Post.

You can connect with him by visiting thebodylogic.com

Disclaimer:

The material provided in this book is for educational and informational purposes only and is not intended as medical advice. The author and publisher of this material are not responsible in any manner whatsoever for any injury that may occur through following the recommendations contained in this material. The information contained in this book/eBook should not be used to diagnose or treat any illness, metabolic disorder, disease, or health problem. If you have developed a serious illness of some kind, the complexities of dealing with such challenges are best handled by your physician or health care provider, whom you should consult with before beginning any nutrition or exercise program. Use of the programs, advice and other information contained in this book/eBook is at the sole choice and risk of the reader.

CONTENTS

1 "One meal to rule them all"

2 Systems the AlphaMeal performs on

3 Hormones & Hormesis

4 Goal specific framework- weight loss, fat loss, muscle gain, brain power

5 What to do if you're not a breakfast person

6 What if you're fasting

7 Eating consistency

8 COFEE, COFFEE, COFFEE

9 A word on water

10 Conclusion

Appendix: Bonus Articles

PART 1
One meal to rule them all

"Make sure you eat your breakfast!!"

Remember when your mom or grandmother or some family member reminded you of the need to eat your breakfast? We usually remember this in the context of it being sort of annoying and some groaning was involved, either because you didn't want to eat, or you didn't get to eat what you really wanted which for me as a kid was cupcakes. Breakfast is just one of those things we were always told to eat and that it was "an important start to the day".

But how? No one ever seemed to be able to explain that part except for the generic you need "energy for the day".......(yawn), gimme something better than that ma or gimme cupcakes!!

Well look no further you'll get the answers you seek and it's not going to be some fluffy public service announcement about how breakfast is important for calories and how you need to "kickstart" your metabolism (although it does that, as well as give you energy for your day so mom wasn't entirely wrong).

You're going to get the real operational dynamics of the meal that **"breaks the fast"** and how it plays a role in health, fitness and performance. No matter if you're an individual just looking to be healthy and well or if you're a high level sports of physique athlete breakfast is a critical to achieving your goals.

"One meal to rule them all"

That statement is more than just a Lord of the Rings reference. Breakfast is the alpha meal for several reasons. First off the morning is the start of a new day biologically speaking. When you wake up in the morning it's like your body is punching in for its shift and it's time to go to work. Multiple biochemical systems and processes are "ramping" up to coincide with the rising of the sun and a state of wakefulness and alertness.

"The prior nights' sleep is a barometer for your productivity, energy and function for the day ahead".

Breakfast is an opportunity to direct your body toward being optimized when you awaken. If you slept terribly you can use breakfast to help mitigate and even correct a crappy night's sleep. If you slept great you can use breakfast to enhance the recovery you got and help you make gains in your health, fitness and overall productivity. It's a win-win.

"Breakfast is a meal that has the ability to make metabolic corrections or enhancements depending on your waking status".

What we're talking about here folks is momentum. "The Alpha meal… breakfast drives biological momentum". An activator, initiator, catalyst. Other meals during the day don't have the same impact to the degree that breakfast does. As I previously mentioned it doesn't matter if you're simply seeking a boost in overall wellness and vitality or you're a high performing athlete, breakfast is the tool to get the job done.

THE COFFEE CONUNDRUM

This is an important topic to cover but I'd like to be clear that coffee is part of the Alpha meal program, and it has its own section. This doesn't mean you have to drink it if you're not a coffee drinker. Coffee is a conditional tool that can be used to enhance the protocols in different ways which we'll go over towards the end. As a tool, with the right metabolics, it can be a powerful aid to hitting your fitness goals. Most people however are not in this category and instead use coffee to make up for massive gaps in energy, focus, productivity and horrible sleep hygiene. If coffee has replaced your metabolism, realize that it's a poor substitute, which is why Native Americans use to refer to it as "empty fire". It can definitely get the job done but in a person that is in a dysfunctional and dependent state with it it's like drinking from a fire hose when you're thirsty. We'll go over some of the negative effects it can have on your body to which you should use a way to self-asses if you over consume and rely on it.

Many people rely on coffee to function. This is not good. Most people realize this is not good, but they're not exactly sure why or how it's not good, hence a little explanation will elucidate and maybe make you reconsider your habits.

When you replace your metabolism with coffee/caffeine it has several affects that you'll notice play out in other aspects of your health and your life. Coffee in a dependent state is actually counterproductive to the three main systems that a proper alpha meal breakfast would optimize (which we'll go over shortly). Coffee does rev your metabolism, it's a stimulant, but it does so artificially, not a good position to be in because you'll always need it. It can further destabilize blood sugar by causing wild swings, especially if you load it up with sugars and syrups. Finally due to the addictive nature of coffee it automatically predisposes you to a rearrangement of your neurotransmitters that reinforces addictive behaviors, and fluctuations in your mood which can drive down creativity and productivity.

Another important point to cover is a principle in biology known as M.E.N.S. It stands for **Minimal Electrical Neuromuscular Stimulation.** This is how metabolic substitution begins when you're reliant on coffee. This principle basically means your body will try to use the least amount of energy for a particular process to satisfy the 1st law of thermodynamics which is the conservation of energy. The more you expose yourself to coffee in quantity, frequency and volume the more you activate the M.E.N.S principle and serve it up on a silver platter. Your biology is basically saying why utilize the processes of energy balance in the body when it's being provided by coffee? Thus the body will down regulate such processes to conserve that energy. This eventually leads to your metabolism essentially getting "out of shape". So when it's time to lose weight, burn fat, perform a workout or play with the kids and you need your metabolism to be operational you can't do it or you're very slow to get going without coffee.

Most people intuitively know if they fit into the category of "non-functional" without caffeine. Just in case you don't, take a day without drinking it and see how you do; a natural drop in energy is par for the course so that doesn't count. If you have 3 or more drops in energy during the day, your metabolism is out of shape.

If you take a day off from coffee and experience headaches, irritability, monkey mind, or an inability to mentally perform even common everyday tasks, it's in your best interest health wise to reduce and/or cycle your coffee consumption. That could be cutting the amount you have in half or even alternating days. Don't go cold turkey because that sets off alarms in your body and it will push back hard. Start small, reduce the ounces you have, get a smaller cup, reduce the amount of cups you have in a day, bracket consumption to the morning only. You can then move on to every other day or every two days. You should be able to function if coffee/caffeine is not present, and you want to get yourself to that point so your metabolic systems can turn back on.

Consider the last few pages a disclaimer and way to self-assess to see where you stand with coffee it's not hard to figure out. If you're on the side of dependence and reliance try to do something about it, it will be in your best interest biochemically and metabolically speaking. Back to our regularly scheduled programming of the Alpha meal and how it's a performance enhancer for all health and fitness goals.

FITNESS GOALS

The Alpha meal program will help you structure and design your breakfast to achieve four primary fitness goals:

-FAT LOSS

-WEIGHT LOSS

-MUSCLE GAIN

-BRAIN POWER

These fitness goals are organized by the most popular. Fat loss is hands down the most popular fitness goal, even if it's not initially stated or expressed by a person. Losing bodyfat is desired by virtually all groups pursuing fitness goals. Weight loss is the 2nd most popular goal with a loss of bodyfat already implied in the process, it's kind of understood. The next goal is muscle gain, lean tissue gain. It's important to understand this is not referring to hypertrophy or "bulk" we're trying to use the alpha meal to achieve increases in lean tissue. The last fitness goal is brain power. Being able to increase your productivity at work or at the gym is important and if you can acquire a higher level of control with it your performance will improve and the Alpha meal can definitely be used to do that.

Each fitness goal will have a framework for you to follow that will help you structure your meal appropriately. Having a framework gives you the ability to make different choices and selections in foods. Following the framework is the protocols. The protocols are the specifics and nutrient targets to help you implement each goal. Getting the Alpha meal on point is a massive step to lining up the rest of your actions, habits and behaviors to achieve our health and fitness goals.

ALPHA MEAL UPGRADES

The Alpha meal not only works directly on several systems of the body it also, with consistency and time can upgrade some of the aspects of your metabolism that are favorable for not only achieving your fitness goals but maintaining them as well. If you take a little time to observe there are certain patterns that are similar to "fit" people versus people who aren't fit. The Alpha meal upgrades performance and three different categories.

THERMOGENIC POWER

One of the things that separates fit and healthy people from the rest is that they have thermogenic power, they can burn calories, and burn them hotter, extract more nutrients from foods and get higher yields from foods. The thermic effect of food, which is the biological cost associated with metabolizing and processing food that results in the burning of calories, heat and water is highly dependent on the food selection. Not all foods have the same thermic effect some are lower and some are higher, you want the higher ones. Thermogenic power is not just about when you eat either it's a physiological state so when you're at home, when you're asleep if you have higher a thermogenic capacity you'll be burning at higher rate than if you were at a lower capacity, this is one of the ways fit people stay fit.

<u>INSULIN OPTIMIZATION</u>

Insulin is a very powerful hormone that does a lot of things, much more than just blood sugar management which is what it's commonly known for. Insulin functions in terms of stability and sensitivity. One of the hallmarks of health and fitness across the board is having insulin function that is stable, sensitive and responsive. Folks that have diabetes, high levels of inflammation, and obesity all exhibit insulin resistance and destabilization at some level. Insulin is crucial to bodyfat levels, immunity, building muscle, burning fat, it's a powerful hormone AND is primarily under our control with the foods we eat and the way we eat them, this is a major key- to have a powerful hormone like this under our control, with others like testosterone, leptin and cortisol we can influence them but we don't have the same level of control like we do with insulin. This is a secret weapon that you can unlock with the Alpha meal.

CIRCADIAN RHYTHM

You may be wondering what's the circadian rhythm have to do with muscle, burning fat and breakfast? Well it has everything to do with it, your body operates on a schedule it has for thousands of years via evolution; this schedule sits on a 24 hour cycle and is tied to the cycles of the sun light and dark. Now this is a complex topic but let's just say a healthy circadian rhythm allows you to get good quality sleep, boosts your anti-oxidant capacity, stay lean and healthy and of course happy which matters. Most people have a jacked up circadian rhythm. Breakfast can help you find that beat and put you back on track , that's what makes it Alpha.

Properly leveraging the alpha meal is like hitting the ground running making it a versatile tool. To understand how versatile a tool breakfast is we have to understand the status or condition the body is in in the morning hours to appreciate the value.

The morning time, besides being a figurative start to a new day, is also a new day or the start of a new biological cycle in a manner of speaking. Your body has the circadian rhythm, the system of clocks operating on a 24 hour cycle. Glands, organs, hormones, metabolism and more synch up to Diurnal (daytime) cycles and nocturnal (night) cycles. They engage in actions such as activity, idling, restoration, and sensitivity. All these patterns are coupled to the 24 hour cycle and have been so evolving over thousands of years hardwiring into human biology.

Your diurnal rhythm or day time is the active state; you're "doing". The nocturnal state is the time to clean up, repair and restore so you can wake up and "do" more the next day. Your ability to "do" is highly contingent upon your ability to repair and rejuvenate. That means sleep needs to be of appropriate quality and quantity to keep the system going.

"Most people today have horrible sleep hygiene: poor in both quality and quantity".

Breakfast is an opportunity to use nutrition to correct poor or inadequate recovery and by the same token used as a performance enhancer when sleep and recovery is adequate. The morning is a crucial time relative to other times of the day because many of our biological systems initiate and ramp up activity in the morning. We will be covering three of the main systems here but your ability to influence these systems with nutrition or the "breakfast meal" is not the same at lunch or dinner. The train is already moving figuratively speaking as the morning progresses and it can become increasingly difficult to optimize yourself as time passes in the day.

PART 2
Systems the Alpha meal performs on

"The Alpha meal has the power to make you go anabolic or get you out of being catabolic"

Breakfast has an operational dynamic as mentioned before. The meal itself is a signaling system to the body. In essence that's what we're actually trying to accomplish; signaling the system to do what we want it to do-be it fat loss, weight loss muscle gain, etc. In this program we're using food as a signal by way of the breakfast meal but the approach can be drilled down to purely signaling even if a traditional "meal" is not feasible for some reason.

It's also important to understand that your food selection or even omitting breakfast sends a signal as well, one that may not be desirable if you're having trouble reaching your goals.

It's important to make the distinction between the "operation" and the "convention". The convention is the tradition of eating breakfast that says we should be eating this "full" meal between the hours of 7 and 9 a.m. Your plate should have a bowl of cereal, eggs, toast, bacon, glass of milk, and a glass of orange juice. These traditions don't necessarily yield the particular operation we're looking for.

The goals for this program are *fat loss, weight loss, lean tissue gains, and brain power output.* The "operation" were looking to achieve is signaling the systems of the body to optimize our physiology to help us reach these goals quicker. The morning time is the greatest position of leverage to do this. The signaling effect we're trying to have comes from that **"first food exposure".** This is the first thing that you ingest which informs and directs the body on how to carry out the patterns of physiology in our systems. The first food exposure is in essence information. This information is processed as soon as a food hits our mouth.

Our physiology has a feedback loop in it known as the neuro-lingual response. This is a loop between the tongue and the brain. When a food or ingredient hits the tongue the neuro-lingual reflex relays the information to the brain and the brain initiates and responds by directing various processes and communicating to other organs in the body about what's going on.

This is why there are certain medications or supplements that are consumed in liquid form. The directions for some meds and liquid supplements recommend holding the ingredient under the tongue to let it dissolve. This amplifies the effect and increases the processing rate of the active ingredients.

The Alpha meal operates on the hardware of the body as well as the software. For the purposes of this program I consider the hardware as systems that run in the background on autopilot, they're always on and make up the undercurrent or foundation of your biology.

The three primary hardware systems that the Alpha meal influences are:

Blood Sugar regulation, Metabolic tone, and Neurotransmitter profile.

I'll be going into these systems in detail shortly. The software of your biology that you have a little more control and influence over are the hormones. Hormones like software interfaces with the hardware. The hardware allows your software to have a place to work, essentially making it run better. This is how you shift your body toward your fitness goals. This is the channel you go through.

Let's take a look at the software features that the Alpha meal has an effect on. *It's important however to remember that the hardware is first, that has to be satisfied before the software (the hormones). The hormones can only work well to the degree that the three hardware systems: Blood Sugar regulation, Metabolic tone, Neurotransmitter profile are optimized.*

Your mother may have not realized or had these systems in mind when she was yelling at you to eat your breakfast but the message is the same. Before we never really understood or explained why it was so important. I'll go into each of these three systems and how they function which will begin to reveal to you the importance of the alpha meal and why it's given this precedence.

BLOOD SUGAR REGULATION

One of the most important systems the Alpha meal has influence over is your blood sugar. The system of blood sugar regulation is important and tightly regulated for a specific reason.

"The most crucial function to any organism is the continuity of the production of energy".

You have to maintain a steady supply of energy in the body to be able to function or you won't survive. We get the raw material and resources to produce energy primarily from food. There are other ways to produce energy such as light and our own physiological processes of metabolism; but for the majority of people; **food is the supply chain.**

The human body developed a sophisticated "thermostat" to monitor and track the status of your supply lines and production of energy. This is your blood-sugar regulation system. Your blood sugar analyzes and forecasts energy production in the short term as well as the long term. Just like a gas light in your car. When your energy production starts to slow down and when the resources or nutrition you have on board to keep the train going diminishes, your gas light comes on. Blood sugar begins to drop and when it gets very low this usually presents symptomatically in the body as lightheadedness, fatigue, nervousness, dizziness, etc.

Blood sugar control has initiatory activity in the morning. There's not really a starting point for blood sugar because it's always on and working, however if any starting point or reset point had to be established it would be in the morning for a few reasons. Energy production and output increases at the start of a new day which is tied to light/dark cycles of the day (circadian rhythm). Also during the prior night's sleep activity is low and blood sugar operationally is running at a low level, you're not eating any food and the body is in a fasting state blood sugar remains relatively quiet. This is why it's called break –fast. When you wake up in the morning blood sugar is typically low, this as well as the other factors I just mentioned make the morning time, "breakfast time" the opportune time to "initiate" and influence activity; when you blood sugar yawns and awakens.

As mentioned before blood sugar runs the spectrum in terms of how it operates. It functions in acute situations as well as chronic ones. A person who is clinically diagnosed as being hypo or hyper glycemic has a blood sugar control problem that is chronic in nature, it's been there for a while and has its own behavior. A person who hasn't eaten over 12 hours for example is going to have very low blood sugar and potentially be symptomatic because energy levels and the resources to build them are extremely low so that person will need to eat. So there are acute situations and chronic ones.

The morning time is crucial because as stated before

"if there is an ideal time to reset or stabilize blood sugar its breakfast".

Your food selection is crucial to optimizing your blood sugar control. The other aspect about blood sugar that a lot of people don't take into in consideration is that it can turn into a runaway train if nutrition is inappropriate. Blood sugar can act like a rollercoaster when you make the wrong nutrition selections. When this happens it can be very difficult to get back on track and can take several hours.

This is why breakfast is crucial, fi you make a poor selection or choose not to eat it can set these rollercoaster conditions off because the morning meal has the most influence. You don't have as much leverage to influence blood sugar control or stabilize it with lunch and dinner or later meals because the train is already moving in a manner of speaking.

Optimizing your blood sugar is one of the keys to being healthy and attaining your fitness goals which we'll go over in detail. It's important to know that optimal blood sugar is stable blood sugar, not high and not low. Obviously blood sugar rises and falls like a tide but a dysfunctional blood sugar looks more like a tidal wave or swell, or a flood or a huge sinkhole. You want it to be stable and respond appropriately, rise then fall, and get back to baseline. There are many symptoms associated with the different states of your blood sugar if it's high, low, or all over the place.

Everyone has a different status on their blood glucose system and if you have more serious, chronic, complicated issues please consult a healthcare professional. For the purposes of the program we'll keep things a little more general. That means some people will have blood sugar that is functional and stabilized while others will be very dysfunctional.

To get a general baseline on your blood sugar status; follow this general assessment.

Upon waking you feel:

-Starving/ ravenous :

Blood sugar is crashing either from a lack of nutrition in terms of time (since you ate last), quality or quantity.

This usually means: **Momentary or chronic destabilization**

-Not hungry for most of the morning:

Blood sugar is relatively stable, and your ability to function is normal without the influence of coffee.

This usually means: **Normal/stable condition**

-Wakeup hungry but dissipates after a short while:

Fairly normal blood sugar control, hunger signal could be a reflex to increased stress or energy demands from exercise or similar factors.

This usually means: **Fairly normal/ under momentary increases in demands.**

-Wakeup and hunger sets in within an hour:

- This is a sign of being fairly normal and stabilized.

This usually means: **Slightly stressed, Fairly normal/stabilized.**

Please remember these guidelines are general and simplified and can change depending on external factors. Everyone will present differently and this baseline assessment is not meant to diminish the complexities of this system, it's a just starting point of reference.

If you experience any or all of these states frequently consider your overall blood sugar destabilized. You may want to examine several factors such as diet, training, sleep, and stress.

The more demand placed on the energy systems of your body via exercise, training, food and stress the more they will influence the behavior and function of your blood sugar control system. This is a dynamic system and it operates differently at different times depending on the circumstances so remember these guidelines are general.

We will go over the specific alpha meal protocols for optimizing blood sugar to achieve our fitness goals. The takeaway points for this system are that your biggest influence is the morning time and it will typically be low from the prior night's sleep.

METABOLIC TONE

The metabolism is very similar to an engine in a car in terms of its abilities and capabilities. Your metabolism is the sum of all processes that take place in the body from the cellular level to a systemic level. For the purposes of simplicity if blood sugar regulation is like the gas light on your car, metabolism is the engine. The metabolism is always on and working with alternating periods of activity and idling. At its lowest output it's still like a car that idles. This is why we refer to it in terms of tone. The "tone" of activity is the highs, lows and all spaces in between depending on the circumstances, but always turned on nonetheless.

Upon waking metabolism is typically in its idle position (generally speaking there are exceptions), after all you've been sleeping all night. The metabolism is typically idling in the morning but that doesn't mean it's been idling all night. While you sleep pulses of metabolic activity occur but for the purposes of this program let's keep the general premise of metabolism;

"that upon waking its idle and the Alpha meal is your opportunity to take it out of neutral and ramp it up."

An optimized metabolism is one that has high power capacity or "horsepower". The higher the horsepower an engine has the greater the capacity. The other feature of an optimized metabolism is high performance. That high powered engine may have a lot of capacity but can it be expressed? Can it perform?

These are two different things here and can be independent of each other. The common inclination is to believe the two are positively correlated when they're not. If you have a high powered metabolism that doesn't necessarily means it performs well. Having a low power metabolism isn't necessarily a bad thing and can be advantageous for various reasons with a low power metabolism you could have great performance and endurance with it.

"For the achievement of most health and fitness goals metabolically you want high power + high performance"

Metabolism is very similar to blood sugar in how it behaves and can be initiated and "kickstarted" in the morning. You can use food or in this case the alpha meal to activate metabolic performance. When you eat food it takes the metabolism out of the idle position and gives it something to churn and crank on. It's important to have a sensitive metabolism that can kick into gear if you're going to achieve any health and fitness goal. If your metabolism can't get out of neutral it makes things very difficult.

Your metabolics is very similar to a fireplace that burns wood or a locomotive that needs a steady supply of coal to move forward. Sleeping and not having anything in the stomach quiets the metabolism like a log that's almost completely burned in a fireplace. There are low level embers but no major fire. Throwing in food is like throwing a fresh log in, turns things on, burns more calories and gives off heat..energy expenditure.

You have to be careful though because you can't just throw any kind of food in and this is what makes the design of the Alpha meal so important. If you throw in a couple of sheets of newspaper into a fire it'll go up in flames immediately and won't provide any sustainability, just a quick burst. If you put on a piece of wood however, the fire will burn all night. The Alpha meal needs to be designed to maximize capacity and performance by stoking a sustainable fire, which you will see in the protocols section utilizing specific macronutrients- protein, carbs and fat.

Metabolism is also similar to blood glucose in that your highest position of leverage is in the morning, another argument for the importance of the Alpha meal. If you don't optimize metabolism at the opportune time it can take a while to kick into gear and you can miss this high activity potential in the morning.

The Alpha meal is also crucial because food selection influences your thermogenic capacity. As just mentioned, the rate at which the metabolic fires crank and grind has a lot to do with the specific macronutrients you eat. You want a high thermogenic capacity to raise your energy expenditure levels to burn at a high level of heat so your body can toast calories. This is also known as the thermic effect of food which is the amount of energy expenditure it requires to complete the transaction of breaking down and digesting foods. Some foods have a higher thermic effect than others and we'll see how that plays a role in the protocols relative to thermogenics and how they pay a role in the specific fitness goals.

NEUROTRANSMITTER PROFILE

Neurotransmitters are becoming more and more popular as more information reveals how much influence they have on the body and the alpha meal can directly affect them. Neurotransmitters are critical to your mood, emotional states, creativity, connection, and overall wellbeing. They are primarily manufactured in the gut and brain and act non-locally throughout the body.

There are many neurotransmitters in the body and people tend to have a particular dominance in one, a sub dominance in another and a more recessive acting one. This is why it's often referred to as a profile. As stated there are many different types of neurotransmitters but we'll focus on the primary ones in this program.

Acetylcholine – Primary activating neurotransmitter responsible for memory, alertness, reaction time and focus.

Dopamine –The feel good chemical involved in pleasure, pattern recognition, "reward" constructs, highly addictive.

Serotonin/Oxytocin- Connection, self-worth, self-awareness, depression, euphoria, creativity, calm.

GABA- Pain reducer, feelings of well-being, world view and perspective, creativity, calm.

Again it's important to reiterate that there are many other neurotransmitters but these are the major ones.

While the characteristics associated with each of these each neurotransmitters above are listed, the amounts and levels that will facilitate the actions of their associated characteristics are different and unique to the individual and further investigation would be needed to find out how specific you need to be to optimize each one.

Neurotransmitter dynamics are multifaceted. They don't really have a rhythm because they activate at different times for different reasons. They have influences on other chemicals and functions in the body.

"They add an accent to biological processes that enriches experience and expression like a well seasoned meal."

For example exercise typically results in a dopamine release directly after. Eating a meal with a close friend or loved one causes a boost in oxytocin. Good quality sleep can boost your serotonin making you feel happier, more motivated and productive.

Sleep is a time when neurotransmitters "charge their batteries" in a sense. As just stated they don't really have a rhythm and are kind of on all the time, either active or dormant depending on the circumstances of the internal and external environment. It's safe to say however that most of the "recharging and reloading" of the neurotransmitters happens during sleep and they're prepped and primed for the next day.

Along with the other two systems your neurotransmitter profile can be leveraged to a high degree using the Alpha meal. The right food selection and macronutrient mix can enhance a desirable profile and help correct a less desirable profile. For example let's say you had a bad day at work which resulted in a poor night's sleep; your serotonin levels may be low which can result in you waking up feeling depressive or in a low energy state. On the other hand you could have had an overproduction of serotonin which can sometimes cause a flow into a very irritable or short tempered state.

Neurotransmitters can be tough to get back into alignment as well if you get off to a bad start. The phrase "woke up on the wrong side of the bed" is the aspect of our biology that that is basically speaking to. The Alpha meal can get in the middle and impact this no matter which side of the bed you woke up on.

Now that we've covered the three main "hardware" systems that the Alpha meal impacts, which if you remember I previously mentioned takes priority over other systems, we can move on to the "software" parts that are impacted by the alpha which are the hormones. There are key hormones that play a big role in our health and fitness goals.

SYNERGISTIC FRAMEWORK

Now that we've covered the important biological systems that the Alpha meal influences; we can see why we've always been told breakfast is so important but may have not been readily aware of.

In case you didn't notice there are common patterns consistent among the three systems. There is a synergistic relationship among them and many of the protocols that address one system will often carry over to the others. It's worth pointing out these patterns:

-Each system has its greatest reset or activation point in the morning.

-Each system tends to carry its morning status into the better part of the day. (Takes longer to get back in synch if they're off to a bad start).

-Each of these systems needs to be balanced and optimized to reach fitness goals faster.

The Alpha meal allows you to get in and manipulate what you need to make your biology and metabolics work for you.

PART 3
Hormones and Hormesis

The main hormones we'll focus on are cortisol and insulin. It's important to understand hormones behave in many different states. They have fluctuating rhythms where at times they're more active than others. Hormones can be triggered by some external factor into shifting their state into surges and suppressions. Hormones also have multifaceted communications between the brain, gland of production and the cells itself. We typically describe these relationships in terms of sensitivity and resistance. It's important to point out that hormones are not light switches they're a little more complex.

Another feature of hormones is the hormetic effect they tend to express. Hormesis is the concept that applies to physiology where a little bit of a biochemical like a hormone has beneficial effects on the body, and where that very same chemical in excessive or chronic amounts has harmful effects. Hormones in particular have this feature associated with them. As a rule of thumb the goal is always to be in the hormetic range which is different for everyone and getting to know your body is the key.

Now that we've gone over that, the two most pertinent hormones to focus on that influence the Alpha meal are Cortisol and Insulin. There are many other hormones at play but these are the key players.

CORTISOL

Cortisol is your chief stress hormone and is one of the most important hormones in the body, has the most agency over the tissues of your body and is the most dynamic. Cortisol is a beneficial hormone in the hormetic range. In small amounts/short bursts cortisol is a fat burner, muscle builder, anti-inflammatory and much more. In excessive amounts however it does the exact opposite causing fat storage, muscle breakdown, and is pro-inflammatory. Given this breakdown we want to leverage the hormetic range as much as possible. In order to do that we must understand what the cortisol behavior looks like.

Cortisol does have its own rhythm that's yoked to your

circadian rhythm or body clock and is diurnally active (day time). Its primed and prepped overnight and remains in a very low dormant state (or at least it's supposed to not always the case) cued to surge in the early morning hours to prepare you for the day typically triggered by early morning light.

Ramping up begins in the morning around 5-6 a.m. The uptick in cortisol continues into lunchtime and starts to level off and wind down as the afternoon progresses; which is when the preparation by the body for rest, recovery and sleep take place.

In addition to the diurnal rhythm, cortisol also responds to the stressors of whatever may be present in the morning hours which are different for everyone. This could be the stress of an argument with a loved one, rush hour traffic, a workout (yes exercise is a form of stress), or lack of nutrition.

It's important to understand that stress is not just emotionally driven. There are all kinds of stress and the body doesn't distinguish the difference accumulating it all in to one big pot. Psychological stress will accumulate as much as an intense workout will. You could be out at a big party having the time of your life but if you stay up all night this is absolutely a stress to the body. What really matters is not trying to eliminate stress, that's not always feasible. What we want to optimize is how we respond, manage and clear that stress which is what really determines how detrimental it will be.

Understanding that our chief hormone, cortisol is active in the morning and is also active to respond to whatever stressors are in our environment, it's easy to see that our cortisol can rack up really quick in the morning. Given this potential scenario it's also realistic to say that it would be really easy to blow right past cortisol's "hormetic range" and put you in a danger zone. For these reasons we want to keep cortisol even keel so we can keep its influence shifting us toward our fitness goals.

INSULIN

Insulin is a very interesting hormone and has many functions in the body. It's one of the most beneficial and essential hormones we have and we have to be careful with it because it can exert quite a lot of power over our physiology. Insulin is anabolic in nature; it brings resources to tissues for synthesis. The hormetics of insulin is a particularly strong feature and leveraging it can have powerful effects. Insulin doesn't have as concrete of a rhythm as cortisol does but as generally it fluctuates throughout the day with a very low activity state overnight during sleep. These patterns though, can and do change with our actions and behaviors.

Just as cortisol has its own trajectory and is influenced by external stressors; insulin in addition to its own rhythm is heavily influenced by food, which means we have a large amount of control over it with our choices in food. Insulin in the hormetic range has many of the same benefits as cortisol; lean tissue building, fat burning, antioxidant and anti-inflammatory. In excessive or chronic amounts this is flipped. We typically see this as insulin resistance or people who have diabetes.

The way we want to approach insulin is to keep it as sensitive as possible to achieve our fitness goals. The more insulin is activated and the more you use it the more desensitized it becomes and you begin to develop resistance where the cells stop responding to it and then you increase the amounts of circulating insulin in the body knocking you out of that hormetic range into the unhealthy zone which is where we don't want to be. Using the Alpha meal to strategically use insulin to your advantage will be shown in the protocols to leverage the benefits as much as possible.

Important note: The landscape of hormonal dynamics (cortisol and insulin in particular) described here are general. It's important to remember that every person has an individuality to their hormonal dynamics that is specific to them based on lifestyle, habits, actions and overall health. If there are more serious issues with your body systems and your hormones consult a healthcare professional.

PART 4

GOAL SPECIFIC FRAMEWORK

Ok here we are what to do for each fitness goal. In this section we'll go over the framework for how you set up and structure your meals to achieve each fitness goal. The framework is a generalized set up; in my professional experiences I've come across many people that just want to be told what to do and what to eat , but that is equivalent to giving a man to fish instead of teaching a man to fish. The intention with outlining the framework is so that you can do this on your own and self-direct to achieve your goals.

FAT LOSS

Fat loss is specifically the loss of fatty tissue particularly White adipose tissue. The main concern is outside of actual bodyweight although it's implied that some weight loss may be associated with this process everyone will respond differently. You may not want to lose any bodyweight, which is to say you want to retain your muscle tissue, but again the specificity is on fat tissue. The framework used here is about optimizing macronutrient ratios and the hormones to make this process happen. Real fat loss is about mobilization; "burning" what we have not what we just ate recently.

What's needed is:

-High level metabolics

-Higher ratios of proteins (predominant macronutrient)

-Moderate fat content

-Low carbohydrate content filling in

the rest of the meal

<u>FAT LOSS NUTRIENT TARGETS</u>:

PROTEIN TARGETS- 3-6 OZ or between 25-40 grams of protein in a serving if you're a bigger individual you want to have a serving size closer to the 6 ounces or the 40 grams; if you're a smaller individual 3 ounces or 25 grams.

CARBOHYDRATE TARGETS- 1-2 cups of veggies or medium glycemic level fruits. We want low sugar foods, this doesn't mean zero sugar foods, just lower. Try to stick with fruits and veggies as options that will eliminate a lot of the poor choices with other types of breakfast "carbohydrate" foods. Ok serving sizes 1-2 cups depending on the food but a normal portion size is good.

FAT TARGETS- 1-2 oz/tablespoons peanut butter, olive oil, coconut oil we're looking at about 1-2oz or tablespoons and it doesn't have to be precise or exact, it doesn't have to count the fat that's in the foods you're eating, it can be in addition to, just don't make it zero fat that's all.

PROTEIN 50%

FAT 30%

CARBS 20%

<u>SAMPLE MEALS</u>

<u>BREAKFAST OPTION #1</u>

-2-3 EGG VEGETABLE OMELET

- VEGETABLES CONSIST OF A SALSA MIX: ¾ CUP MIX OF ONIONS, GREEN AND RED PEPPERS, TOMATOES

-BREAKFAST MEAT: BACON, CANADIAN BACON, TUKEY BACON, SAUSAGE, NUTS, ETC.

BREAKFAST OPTION #2

-SMOKED SALMON

-2 POACHED EGGS

-BOWL OF CHOPPED TOMATOES, RED ONIONS, CUCUMBERS

-SMALL CAPPUCCINO

BREAKFAST OPTION #3

-½- 1 ½ CUPs QUINOA

-2-3 TABLESPOONS CRUSHED ALMONDS ON TOP

-1 TABLESPOON COCONUT OIL

-DASH OF SEA SALT AND CINNAMON

-2-3 SLICES OF TEMPEH (FAKIN BACON)

<u>WEIGHT LOSS</u>

This particular goal is specifically geared toward dropping bodyweight, we're not as concerned about dropping bodyfat here but of course it's implied and is built into the framework. The process of losing bodyweight versus purely bodyfat are slightly different but rest assured fat will be burned too. Losing weight is about a shift in physiology not just a diet and not just exercise. It's an ensemble of factors. Meals should be structured for a calorie cut between 100-400 calories per day to initiate weight loss.

<u>*What's needed is:*</u>

-High level metabolics

-Higher ratios of proteins (predominant macronutrient)

-Moderate carbohydrate content

-Lower fat filling in the rest of the meal

- A caloric reduction between 100-400 calories per day, (depending on how much weight you want/need to lose). Do this gradually over time, don't do a sharp drop give yourself a few days or even a week or two.

WEIGHT LOSS NUTRIENT TARGETS

PROTEIN TARGETS- 3-6 OZ or between 25-40 grams of protein in a serving if you're a bigger individual you want to have a serving size closer to the 6 ounces or the 40 grams; if you're a smaller individual 3 ounces or 25 grams.

CARBOHYDRATE TARGETS- 1-2 cups of veggies or medium glycemic level fruits.

FAT TARGETS- 1-2 oz/tablespoons peanut butter, olive oil, coconut oil

PROTEIN 50%

CARBS 30%

FAT 20%

SAMPLE MEALS

BREAKFAST OPTION #1

3-6 OZ LEAN CHICKEN (BREAST)

1 ½ CUPS OF STIR FRY VEGGIES

1-2 TABLESPOONS OF TOASTED SESAME OIL OR COCONUT OIL

1 SMALL APPLE

BREAKFAST OPTION #2

3-6 OZ BACON

1 ½ CUP OF STEAMED BROCCOLI

1 GRAPEFRUIT

BREAKFAST OPTION #3

2 HARD BOILED EGGS

½ LARGE AVOCADO

FRESH SQUEEZED LEMON JUICE

2-3 DASHES OF SEA SALT

BREAKFAST OPTION #4

KALE SALAD- SLICED APPLES, CUCUMBERS, PUMPKIN SEEDS, HANDFUL OF WALNUTS, HANDFUL OF ALMONDS, BALSAMIC VINAIGRETTE.

MUSCLE GAIN

The goal of muscle gain is to specifically add lean tissue to your frame, not bulk up. Putting on muscle is more a function of how you train otherwise a person could just bulk up by eating more protein but it doesn't really work that way. Weight gain or lean tissue gain just as it is weight loss is a result of an ensemble of factors. So the nutritional recommendations here will support the environment for whatever lean tissue changes you're stimulating via training.

Meals should be structured for a calorie increase between 100-300 additional calories per day, gradually over the course of a few days or weeks. cortisol slightly peaked above normal around training if possible but otherwise stable. Finally an insulin spike at the Alpha meal and post training is recommended.

What's needed is:

-Higher ratios of proteins (predominant macronutrient)

-Selective/Low-Moderate carbohydrate content

-Lower fat filling in the rest of the meal.

- A caloric increase between 100-300 calories per day, (depending on how much weight you want/need to lose). Do this gradually over time, don't do a sharp increase give yourself a few days or even a week or two.

-Cortisol quiet but spiked during training.

-Insulin spiked, especially during training.

MUSCLE GAIN NUTRIENT TARGETS:

PROTEIN TARGETS- 4-7 OZ

CARBOHYDRATE TARGETS- 1/2-1 cup of medium glycemic carbohydrate (between 30-60 on the chart) 1 cup of high fiber veggies.

FAT TARGETS- 1-2 oz/tablespoons peanut butter, olive oil, coconut oil.

PROTEIN 40%

CARBS 40%

FAT 20%

SAMPLE MEALS

BREAKFAST OPTION #1

4 SCRAMBLED EGGS

½ CUP QUINOA SEASONED WITH OLD BAY, SEA SALT

1 CUP OF GREEN BEANS

BREAKFAST OPTION #2

2 CUPS OF GROUND TURKEY,

½ LARGE SWEET POTATO

1 ½ CUP OF VEGGIES

1 TBSP BUTTER (ON SWEET POTATO)

BREAKFAST OPTION #3

½ CUP BLACK BEANS OR LENTILS
½ CUP JASMINE RICE
1-2 CUPS OF HIGH FIBER VEGGIES

BRAIN POWER OUTPUT

Ok let's talk brain power, the goal here is to specifically improve your brain output, give you clarity, improve thinking, creativity and overall productivity. This is obviously a non-traditional fitness goal but the brain is as much of a muscle that needs to be worked and properly fueled as any other muscle in your body. The brain is also critical for your nervous system and performance as well as your mental/emotional capacity which plays a role in training drive and motivation. We're looking for good quality fats and proteins with very low sugar content.

What's needed is:

-Higher ratios of proteins (predominant macronutrient)

-Moderate fat content

-Ultra low carbohydrate filling in the rest of the meal.

BRAIN POWER NUTRIENT TARGETS:

PROTEIN TARGETS- 3-6 OZ

CARBOHYDRATE TARGETS- 1 ½ cups of high fiber veggies

FAT TARGETS- 1-2 oz/tablespoons peanut butter, olive oil, coconut oil

PROTEIN 50%

FAT 30%

CARBS 20%

SAMPLE MEALS

BREAKFAST OPTION #1

Grass fed ground beef

Two tablespoons of ground almonds (mixed in the burger)
1 ½ cup tomato/cucumber salad w/

Tablespoon olive oil

BREAKFAST OPTION #2

Ground turkey w/
Handful of sliced almonds

heaping tablespoons of salsa mix

all in a bowl.

BREAKFAST OPTION #3

Baked tilapia 4- 6 ounces

Apple walnut salad – apples, walnuts, lettuce, cucumbers, balsamic vinaigrette

PART 5
WHAT TO DO IF YOU'RE NOT A

"BREAKFAST" PERSON

This is a big topic here because everyone has different habits and behaviors some people are just not the "breakfast" type but that doesn't mean you still can't take advantage of the alpha meal. You absolutely can even if breakfast isn't your thing.

In my experiences over the years I find that people typically fall into one or more of these 4 scenarios if they're not the breakfast type:

Can't eat first thing in the morning

This is you if your stomach is just not ready 1st thing, you have no taste for food and if you do eat or sometimes even think about eating first thing in the morning you might get nauseous.

"I can't eat a full meal for breakfast"

You can eat in the morning but not like a big meal or anything you just don't have the appetite or you feel gross if you have a big ol breakfast.

"I usually don't eat breakfast until later in the morning"

You're the type of person that will eat breakfast just later like when you get to work or something or just not when you first wake up or anything like that.

I'm not a "breakfast" person

You've never really been a person that eats breakfast you typically skip it. Not a huge fan of the conventional "breakfast" foods, you pretty much just go right to lunch or you may have a coffee and a health bar or something or a smoothie.

If you fall into any one of these categories it's not really a problem you can still leverage the alpha meal and take advantage of this to reach your fitness goals.

1st off the Alpha meal is really not so much about the meal proper, its' really about the opportunity we have in the morning to make corrections, optimize things and improve our biological performance and we can do this with the first meal/ morning meal which we've come to call breakfast, so it's like a tool. The foods we select to make up a meal are intended to signal to our body, all of the systems we're trying to influence, moving us closer to our goals of fat loss, weight loss, muscle gain etc. A "signal" can be sent with a small amount of food, a drink or even a supplement if you do it right. If you want to spike insulin you can use a granola bar, if you wanted to fire up your metabolism a hardboiled egg works. If breakfast isn't your thing that's cool what you really need is the signaling, you don't have to do a full on meal.

Now it's important to mention the healthier and more fit you are the more you can get away with this "signaling" approach as opposed to the meal, generally speaking. But the less healthy you are, or the harder it's been for you to reach your goals, an actual meal becomes more important, effective and advantageous to improve your function and get you closer to your goals. This is a very important point, and is the best starting answer to the question of whether you need to eat breakfast. If you're healthy and fit you can get away with skipping it, if you're not it becomes more important to eat it.

Now I do realize that some of you may be thinking if I can just signal the system and forego the meal, why not just do that? Why take in extra calories if you don't have to? Great thought, but here's the problem with that… to a certain degree caloric adequacy is part of the equation for all the fitness goals you're looking to achieve. Depending on your personal situation calories are actually important to facilitate the process of weight loss, fat loss or even weight gain. You need them to burn more and burn hotter. This point often flies over people's heads, oftentimes we try to reduce calories to lose fat and weight which only works to a certain point before the body puts the brakes on. If you don't put in enough wood to keep the fire going it will burn slow and low and then when you do put some wood in it will sit because the fire is too weak. I've seen many people do this and it sets them back massively. As a general rule of thumb the more difficult it's been to reach your goals or the less healthier you are eating an actual meal becomes a more effective strategy.

For the people that are concerned about eating a full-on meal; piggybacking off of the signaling approach you don't have to as long as you get the right signals from an appropriate "snack" or small bite of something.

Another point is timing. Timing doesn't have to be specific it's not like if you wake up at 6:30 in the morning you have to eat breakfast by 6:45. The Alpha meal is a window that falls in the morning. Ideal times are between 7am and 9. So it doesn't have to be first thing.

And for you breakfast skippers. Skipping may be the very thing that's preventing you or slowing you down in reaching your goals. Skipping breakfast and waiting until lunch can sometimes short change you because a lot of the systems; your metabolism, blood sugar, and neurotransmitters settle into their rhythm within about a half hour of waking sometimes more sometimes less and depending on sleep, stress, etc this could be a good rhythm or a bad one. Your ability to use breakfast, the alpha meal, as a way to correct a bad body rhythm or enhance a good one decreases the later you put off that first meal. If you're the type of person that doesn't eat until lunch you most likely have missed the boat and probably are running off of caffeine in some way shape or form or pure stress or both which equals bodyweight and fat gain over extended periods of time.

PART 6: WHAT IF YOU'RE FASTING?

Fasting is a popular approach that more and more people are experimenting with. Fasting has numerous health benefits and is a topic for another program in and of itself. There are many ways and methods of fasting and regardless of which one you're using the alpha meal approach in this situation can still be utilized. The approach here is "first food exposure" or "signaling". If you're fasting for extended periods of time especially during the morning hours your "signaling" approach can simply come from a supplement or a drink. For example a couple of BCAA (branched chain amino acids) and a green tea is a potent signal for fat burning and assisting with your workout and muscle tissue. You can implement the same kind of strategy if you're doing a phasic fast within a 24 hour day. The most popular is 16:8, where you fast for 16 hours and eat in an 8 hour window. Phasic fasting is adjustable as long as you adhere to your specific time window for eating and for fasting. A lot of people choose to fast in the morning and leave their eating window for the afternoon into the evening. It's definitely more convenient and easy to do however if we go back to the principles discussed earlier about the importance of breakfast and the morning time as being a prime opportunity to capitalize and influence multiple systems in your biology we can apply the same rule of thumb I just gave. The less healthy you are the more important breakfast becomes. If you're coming from an unhealthy place and decide to use phasic or intermittent fasting as a strategy to improve health, you will typically find more success by keeping your feeding times in the morning and fasting times in the evening. The reason for this is because if you're coming from an unhealthy place it's safe to say that some of your systems are off and this makes breakfast more influential, you'll be able to meet your goals quicker and has a more positive effect on your circadian rhythm and many other systems.

PART 7 : EATING CONSISTENCY:

One of the things that's important to remember is that part of eating is not only to enjoy but also to produce an outcome. Most people forget the outcomes part. Too many people view their nutritional approach as a form of entertainment in taste appearance, variety, etc.

A whole other book could be written about this subject alone but we'll focus on the aspect of eating consistently. Eating the same foods everyday has some merits to it. It adds a level of stability which is one of the precursors the body seeks out whenever you're trying to make changes. This is why a lot of people fail at diet and exercise because the body hasn't gotten the green light from stability in order to justify and authorize a change. As I mentioned earlier fat loss, weight loss, muscle gain happen from an ensemble of factors that shift your biology to that end. If you exercise and diet for 3 weeks straight then get off track for another 2 weeks then get back on, the body will stop responding to that inconsistency. It won't make the investment. While eating the same thing every day can be a tad boring, again it will add a level of stability that will make reaching your goals easier. You also have to consider that if you've had difficulty reaching your goals in the past there's some level of instability and/or metabolic resistance that may need to be rehabbed through the approach of consistent eating that the body can rely and depend on. Whenever I work with people who metabolically teeter I have them eat the same things everyday for a period of time to settle things down.

PART 8: COFFEE, COFFEE, COFFEE

Coffee; What's its place and how does it fit in to the Alpha meal?

At the beginning of the book I outlined the dangers of coffee if you're addicted to it. If coffee has become your new metabolism and new agent of "function" you basically have to de-zombify yourself. Some people can't function at all unless they're caffeinated all day long; not a good system. If you're in a good place with coffee, however and you two are getting along you can leverage this powerful tool when you use it wisely.

Some of the positive factors to coffee are:

FAT BURNING- Caffeine shuttles fatty acids into the bloodstream for energy

PERFORMANCE ENHANCER- Coffee is an adenosine inhibiter which is the component that causes brain fatigue and breakdown.

PAIN RESPONSE- Coffee blunts the pain response allowing you to perform for longer and have more tolerance.

HUNGER SUPPRESSOR – Coffee has compounds in it known as cholinomimetics that can curb hunger which is conditionally useful.

Drinking coffee is pretty synergistic with all of the fitness goals laid out here with some slight adjustments. To put out a few guidelines on consumption it's best to drink coffee as plain as possible. If you put in tons of cream and sugar and syrups it's not a coffee drink anymore it turns more into the equivalent of an ice cream sundae. Also people metabolize caffeine differently, some are rapid metabolizers and others are slower. The faster the metabolization the more careful you have to be because it can wire your nervous system making you jittery, giving you anxiety, and reduce your ability to focus. These same conditions can occur if you drink coffee later in the day as well. Drinking coffee if you're sensitive enough will cause the same symptoms and make it difficult for you to fall asleep. For all these reasons its best to reduce your coffee consumption to only what you need and drink earlier in the day. Try not to drink coffee after lunchtime so that it has plenty of time to work through your system and clear out. Again this is if you're sensitive and a rapid metabolizer, there are some people who do fine with caffeine and while it's still recommended from an overall health standpoint to consume it in the morning and only in amounts that you need, some people will just have a little more wiggle room than others.

In the past few years everyone has been "hacking" coffee using atypical ingredients to "upgrade" the most popular beverage in the world with the popular "bulletproof" coffee leading the way. Before bulletproof became publicized I was experimenting with it for a year. There are definitely some benefits to drinking coffee with certain "enhancements" in it. Some of these hacks are new and some are very old. One of the reasons why these hacks are worth giving a try is because they do indeed have the potential to provide added benefits and enhance things due to coffee/caffeine being a great carrier, transporter and activator. Coffee can carry agents like MCT oil (medium chained triglycerides) into the brain giving you a burst of energy. Coffee can transport an agent like curcumin across the gut/liver barrier and help and improve its anti-inflammatory effect. Caffeine activates the nervous system and taking something like fish oil with it can improve your performance in the gym. It's these qualities that make hacking coffee worth a shot. I have a bonus product called Coffee Hacks which is a recipe list of various coffee combinations that enhance metabolism, increase fat burn and many more. If you purchased this book you can get the coffee hacks for free, which also include the recommended recipes that are synergistic with each health and fitness goal of the Alpha meal, all you need to do is email the receipt and I'll send it right out to you.

PART 9: A WORD ON WATER

Water is the alpha and omega when it comes to a solution and medium for all biochemical processes in the body. That means you can't even begin to access your health and fitness goals and even access the tissues you're selecting such as fat tissue and muscle without being adequately hydrated. Water is obviously an essential nutrient and most people know of the importance of hydration yet many fail to actually hydrate themselves. Drinking water is something that you should do for all protocols. In order to influence and change the state of the various tissues in your body, these tissues need to be hydrated. Water acts as a transport and carrier as well as medium for virtually all tissues. You can't access your fat cells to burn and liberate their components without water. You can't influence your muscle tissue to grow or even perform one hundred percent unless they're hydrated. In the movies we see scenes where someone is going to start a fire and the first thing they do is douse the fire with a gasoline tank, saturating everything in the area then they light the match. When it comes to upgrading the tissues of your body water functions in the same manner. You have to douse those tissues with water before you can light the match which in this case would be exercise and nutrition. This is how you influence the tissues in your body and make changes quicker. Make sure you drink water first thing in the morning and you can have some with your Alpha meal of course.

Muscle is primarily water and if you want to build it and keep it you must stay hydrated. Fat tissue has less circulation and accessibility so it's important to drink even more if you want to access it to burn it.

Don't drown yourself in fluid especially around eating because it can dilute your digestive juices and enzymes but drink an appropriate amount. As far as hydration needs drink about half your bodyweight in ounces per day. If you're unhealthy or even sick increase that amount.

Water Hack: A trick that a lot of physique and sport athletes use is to drink water in the morning with a pinch of sea salt and squeezed lime juice. This helps with hydration and electrolyte balance and improves access to the cells of your tissues. Drink this mixture in the morning and then switch out to lemon in the afternoon obviously not too much lemon unless you like your water sour and you don't have to add the salt either.

PART 10: CONCLUSION

Ok we're at the end of the road here. I hope you're more informed about the importance of this meal. It may seem like we covered a lot of material and we did but to actually implement this properly is low maintenance. The framework for how you can design your own meals is here as well as sample meals that work well with each protocol. It's important to understand that this book isn't a recipe or cookbook. If you're a foodie or interested in trying different ideas with breakfast utilize the framework in this book and apply it to whatever recipe you find.

To summarize the concept of breakfast it's an important tool that can be utilized for the various jobs in the realm of health and fitness. To end the discussion of whether or not it's important to eat breakfast; it depends. As a general rule of thumb the less healthy you are the more important breakfast becomes in order to make biological corrections and move you toward health (provided the food selection is appropriate). The healthier you are the more you can get away with not eating breakfast. Notice I didn't say you don't need to eat it or it becomes less important. Because of all the systems it influences breakfast will always have importance which is what makes it the Alpha meal.

Thank you for reading this book! If you're interested in more content you can purchase the Alpha Meal Kit which is a program that includes videos, tutorials and demonstrations of me cooking the meals laid out in this book. You of course get this book along with the Alpha Meal kit and if you happened to purchase this by itself you won't be paying twice for the book if you purchase the Alpha Meal Kit as long as you furnish a copy of your receipt for this book.

Also if you're a high powered athlete or competitor I have an advanced level of the Alpha meal- Hyper Alpha Kit which has advanced strategies for performance, conditioning and body composition at an athletic level, be sure to check that out!

APPENDIX: BONUS ARTICLES

If you want to be fit don't screw this meal up!

If you have any sort of health and fitness goals, usually you try to eat in a way that helps you meet those goals, right!?

But let's be honest do you really know if the meal you just ate is getting you any closer to your goal? What about the next one; and the one after that?

Real talk: Most people eat what they "feel" is considered healthy and hope it all works out.

We do this partially because of a lack of education and/or mis-education on the *function of a meal:* what it's supposed to do & how it fits into a healthy lifestyle.

Meals have a functional purpose you can actually put them to work to your advantage.

Ironically the one meal you don't want to screw up is the one most people do; and that's breakfast. You may be thinking you're gonna hear some public service announcement from your grandmother pointing her finger at you about how it's important to eat your breakfast everyday

ummm no you-don't-understand.

Breakfast is the alpha meal, a high performance meal; much more so than lunch or dinner. If you have health and fitness goals at any level basic to advanced....., if you're not dialing in breakfast that's not only like bringing a knife to a gunfight you're also leaving the machine gun you forgot you have at home.

Breakfast is a gear shifter to your body, if done right it helps you to:

-Burn bodyfat

-Lose weight

-Gain muscle

-Increase performance and productivity

It does this by influencing, activating, and revving up multiple systems in the body that typically have their prime window of opportunity for function in the morning.

We all have body clocks right and they typically refresh themselves after overnight sleep, this is the closest thing we have to a reset without our body actually turning off. So when we start a new day we kind of start "fresh". Starting a new day also means being able to get through the day and the body knows that. To get through the day you need 3 major systems primed and ready to go:

-**Metabolic tone** – *This is like the engine in the car, metabolism needs to be turned on and warmed up before you drive.*

-**Blood sugar control**- *This is like the gas in the car, maintenance of blood sugar levels is critical to continuity of energy.*

-**Neurotransmitter profiling**- *this is like driver in the car- healthy neurotransmitters will help your productivity, mood and executive function.*

Guess what all these systems, which are primed and ready to get you going in the morning are contingent upon? ......yeah **FOOD**

This is why breakfast is the alpha meal, you don't really get an opportunity to make this up at lunch and dinner.

That trains left the station, you have no better opportunity to kick the tires and light the fires in your body than at breakfast.

You don't want to screw this up folks but like I said earlier most people do. The alpha meal has leverage, it's got pull it can help you bust through plateaus, burn fat, add lean tissue, help you lose weight, get the dial moving, make you feel healthier, look healthier and be way more productive and energized. You have to pick the right foods and line them up with your goals.

3 ways to get fat in the morning that most people are already doing

The morning is a prime time nutritional opportunity, it's where the alpha meal does its work and earns its name, it gives hints and clues in the word... **break-fast** .

The way most people do breakfast however sabotages goals of losing weight burning bodyfat, putting on muscle or even having a clear mind. If you didn't know any better breakfast in a country like America, breakfast might as well be dessert. There's mismatched macronutrients and inferior food selections.

Here's your 3 point checklist to avoid getting fat and staying healthy and in shape.

Skipping breakfast- Skipping breakfast is not a game rookies can play. What I mean by that is skipping breakfast is actually not a bad practice and under the right circumstances it can be a very healthy and powerful tool but if and only if you have the right metabolics for it. What are the right metabolics? A favorable bodyfat percentage (better than the average person) is a robust and strong metabolism, at a maximized capacity for fat burning. If you're struggling with these things and not reaching your goals breakfast is your friend. Breakfast helps to reset, augment and maximize your metabolic activity, blood sugar control and neurotransmitter profile; all crucial systems to reach any of your health and fitness goals and at a crucial time period these systems are no more primed than in the morning after overnight sleep which is why it is the alpha meal. If you want maximize health and greatly up your chances of crushing your fitness goals don't leave this meal on the table.

Eat the wrong breakfast- Hopefully I've convinced you on the merits of actually eating breakfast which is the first step, however for those that already eat it great, but we now have to ask if your selection is appropriate. While there are many systems that breakfast helps to maximize we'll focus on the 3 I just mentioned. It would make sense that if these 3 systems are key to hitting fitness goals it would make sense to eat in a way that optimizes them, right? For metabolic activity we want it high, so eating foods that crank the metabolism and are more thermogenic to up the calorie burn is ideal. For blood sugar control we want that to be stabilized as opposed to yo-yo'ing all over the place, so being mindful of not only the amount sugar we consume in a meal but also the speed at which it enters our body and bloodstream. Finally neurotransmitter profile which is responsible for your productivity, focus and drive needs to be up to par so eating foods that are complete in nature and nutrient dense are ideal versus processed foods. Take a look at what people eat at large as well as yourself to see if you line up with these parameters.

Use coffee as an artificial metabolism – This one is big. America is a caffeinated nation and is the number one legal drug in the world. Coffee is very similar to the first concept just mentioned with skipping breakfast. As a tool, with the right metabolics, it can be a powerful aid to hitting your fitness goals. Most people however are not in this category and instead use coffee to make up for massive gaps in energy, focus, productivity and horrible sleep hygiene. If coffee has replaced your metabolism, realize that it's a poor substitute, which is why Native Americans use to refer to it as *"empty fire"*. It can definitely get the job done but in a person that's in a dysfunctional and dependent state it's like drinking from a fire hose when you're thirsty. Coffee is counterproductive to the three main systems that a proper alpha meal breakfast would instead optimize. Coffee does rev your metabolism... why? because it's a stimulant but if you don't have metabolic control revving it up is against your self interest. It can further destabilize blood sugar by causing wild swings, especially if you load it up with sugars and syrups. Finally due to the addictive nature of coffee it automatically predisposes you to a rearrangement of your neurotransmitters that reinforces addictive behaviors which can drive down creativity and productivity if you're not careful.

Bottom line here is the further away you are from your health and fitness goals no matter what experience or level you are the more necessary and valuable the Alpha meal becomes. The closer you are to your goals and the more optimized your system is the more you can actually leverage and get away with skipping breakfast, going off track with food selection and using coffee to your advantage. Getting there isn't difficult but the foundational value of eating breakfast is one of your most powerful tools to help you achieve your goals.